Keto Done Right
The Ultimate Guide to Real Success on the Keto Diet

Eloise Richards

ELOISE RICHARDS

Contents:

Keto Done Right

The Ultimate Guide to Real Success on the Keto Diet

INTRODUCTION

Welcome to 'Keto Done Right', the only keto meal prep and recipe guide for beginners that teaches you how to actually succeed with the keto diet as opposed to the many who fail. In this book, you'll be shown where most people go wrong and how to prevent weight coming back and prevent getting into bad habits. Essentially, you'll be taught how to keep those pounds off and off for good! What's more is that you'll be guided through tips and tricks that experts in the field of nutrition have contributed to the secret of ketosis. But before we get into all that fabulous stuff, first things first - let's talk about the keto diet, what it is and precisely why it is different.

You might be thinking exactly what I used to think: that keto is just another fad diet that will come and go like every other diet out there that you've heard of a million times. I ask that you remain open-minded because it will be very evident to see that the ketogenic diet is not only NOT a fad diet but one which is backed up by science and nutritionists all across America, the UK, Australia and Europe. The beauty of keto-ing is that it is completely adaptable to the foods you love and unlike other popular diets out there, keto is not a restrictive one. That is, you won't go hungry by cutting thousands of calories from your weekly diet like many erroneous diets teach. Instead, think of keto as the diet that rearranges the foods you already eat into proportions that benefit your body and lead to quick and mostly effective weight loss. If you're still skeptical by the end of this book, all I ask is that you try keto for just a week. Of course, there is only so much weight you can lose in 7 days, however, I promise you that you will feel better, have more energy and be on your way to a much healthier overall lifestyle.

Let's talk a bit about the way we eat nowadays compared to what our bodies really crave, need and do. The modern-day diet and lifestyle are incredibly different from the healthy one that was followed by our ancestors. They suffered from fewer diseases and led long and healthy lives. The rates of modern diseases like obesity and type 2 diabetes were just a fraction of what they are now. These days, people lead a very unhealthy lifestyle and consume too many processed, unhealthy foods. Most people struggle with weight issues and fail to lose extra weight even when they try. Hence, they are all looking for a solution that will show real results. Commonly known as the keto diet, the ketogenic diet has become very popular as of late and is followed by people around the globe. This book will help you understand what the diet is and why people choose to follow it.

As aforementioned, some of you might think that this is just another fad diet that won't work. However, that is far from the truth. This is one of those rare diets that don't require you to fast or starve yourself, go on liquids, or eat tiny, unsatisfying portions. The best part is there is no calorie counting required either. The only prerequisite for the keto diet is that you make a significant reduction in the number of carbohydrates in your diet while you increase the consumption of fats. This might seem unnatural for people who want a diet to lose weight. You might wonder how you will lose fat when you eat more fat. However, this is precisely what the keto diet will help you do.

As you read on, you will understand how this works. You will also get a basic idea of the many ways in which the keto diet can benefit your health and overall well-being. This book will help you understand ketosis, the keto diet, and how you can make it work for you. The recipes in the book will help you get a head start if you decide to follow the keto lifestyle. You will notice that you get to eat a lot of delicious food, even while you lose weight and get healthier.

Why '*Keto*'?

In many ways, I can honestly say that this is the book that I wish I had been able to access when I started out. I hope you are as excited as I was when I first to embarked on my ketogenic lifestyle. That was in 2016, and I haven't looked back. As cliche as it might sound, I was miserably overweight and in-evitably, unhappy. Perhaps like many other folks out there, I had tried every diet you can name and noth-ing worked. I was even exercising properly! That's when I knew I had to take action, and fast. There was no two ways about it. Either I lose weight and start to live healthily or my quality of life would deteriorate further and beyond repair. For a while, I was doing fine with traditional strategies - namely cutting out foods that I loved while pushing my body to its absolute limit with endless cardio sessions. That lasted six months and around Christmas time, my body's natural tendencies caught up with me. I knew that I had no chance in beating my cravings. So, I visited a nutritionist - something I had put off for years and years but her advice changed my life and it is going to transform yours too! She told me to look into keto-dieting and when I asked what it was, she put it to me this way:

'Keto is the diet that changes you into a fat burner'.

What did she mean by this? In today's world, we are surrounded by high sugar, high carb snacks and fast food. The fats we eat are saturated and not the natural kind found in lean meats, nuts and fruit.

From candy bars to easy fries and burgers, our bodies have become used to burning through sugar like it's paper. What the keto lifestyle does however is rewires your metabolism into burning fat the right way. To do this, we readjust our nutritional intake, that is, the food we eat. So what does keto involve exactly?

To put it into simple terms, your diet needs to be centred around:

- High Fat (unsaturated) - 80-150 g
- Medium/Adequate Protein (lean) - 80 - 150 g
- Low Carbohydrate - no more than 60 g

This is the keto motto and the three rules you must live by. Follow them, even vaguely and you will see a difference in your livelihood. However, for the best results, it's important to have meal plans in place as well as a deeper understanding of what foods are good and bad for keto success. In the next chapter, we will be looking at what a keto kitchen looks like and what ingredients make for a tastier and healthier mealtime. Before we get into that, you should be aware that there are three kinds of ketogenic diet.

1. **SKD** (standardized ketogenic dieting)

This is the kind of keto that this book focuses on since it is the easiest to maintain long term and doesn't involve rigid timing, excessive pre-planning and a stressful way of eating.

2. **CKD** (cyclical ketogenic dieting)

Cyclic/cyclical keto is a form of ketogenic diet that involves ratios and distributing what you eat on certain days. One popular form of CKD is where you eat a high carb diet for three days in a week and then for the next two days, you eat no carbs and high protein. While this works for some people, I'm pretty sure you simply don't have the time to be structuring dieting like that. Besides, it often doesn't work long term since we are aiming for a sustainable diet and in effect, a sustainable lifestyle that will keep the pounds off and improve health.

3. **TKD** (targeted ketogenic dieting)

Finally, we have targeted keto dieting. This diet works for those who workout on a consistent basis. With targeted keto, your diet varies depending on when you workout and for how long. You essentially modify your carb intake around the duration of your exercise routine. Again, I would not particularly recommend this one to everyone because it does not enable you to ween off of carbs in a durable way.

--

In essence, SKD (standardized ketogenic dieting) is our goal and to achieve it, we need to ensure that every meal and snack keeps the high-fat, low carb ratio that leads to mind blowing results. If you need more convincing about keto, here are some of the key health benefits to the diet:

-**Lower risk of heart disease.**

-**Lower cholesterol levels.**

-**Reduced risk of some forms of cancer.**

-**Prevents the onset of Alzheimer's disease and dementia.**

-**Decreases epilepsy in children.**

-**Lower risk of Parkinson's disease.**

-Lower levels of insulin.

-Rejuvenation of skin.

-Prevention of type 2 Diabetes.

Ketosis?

So what is ketosis? Ketosis is a metabolic state in the body where fats are burned for energy. This ketosis is induced when the body does not have enough carbohydrates to meet its energy requirements. The natural tendency of any human body is to burn carbs first to provide energy. When the carbohydrate consumption is reduced in the keto diet, the body turns toward fats. It will burn the fat you consume and the fat that is already stored in your body. Carbs provide the easy-to-burn glucose that your body generally uses to gain energy.

When you stop consuming carbohydrates, your body is denied the glucose it needs. This is when it switches to its fat-burning mode. The body shifts to ketosis, and the stored fat is converted to ketones, which are used as fuel by the body. Usually, the body will refrain from burning this fat in the adipose tissues when it undergoes glycolysis. However, under ketosis, the body quickly works on burning this excess fat. This is why other carbohydrate-rich diets cannot help you lose that extra fat, no matter how hard you try.

The increased levels of insulin will block the release of these fats. The keto diet works the opposite way and helps you meet your weight loss goals. Ketosis is how the body adapts to a low carbohydrate environment and allows your body to survive. To induce this state of ketosis, you have to eat the right keto-friendly foods and ensure the proportion recommended for each of the macros. You should be consuming 70 percent fats, 25 percent proteins, and only 5 percent of your diet should be in the form of carbohydrates. The diet can be adjusted to suit personal needs and preferences. For instance, athletes usually increase the number of carbs they consume because they burn it off fast.

The following information will allow you to understand what you should and should not be eating on the ketogenic diet.

Foods You Can Eat on the Keto Diet

Here is a list of foods that you are allowed to eat while on the keto diet:

* Non-starchy vegetables. Eat more of leafy green vegetables. Add some kale, spinach, lettuce, etc. to your grocery list. Also include veggies like cucumber, zucchini, and asparagus. Eat more of the vegetables that grow above the ground and less of

what grows below. Having different vegetables allows you to add variety to your meals.

   * Protein from grass-fed and pastured animal meat such as beef, poultry, and pork. Eggs should also be sourced from such animals. Meat should be consumed in a moderate amount because it can contribute too much protein to your body otherwise. This protein can also be converted to glucose by the body, and it can prevent ketosis.

   * Healthy fats from ghee, lard, coconut oil, chicken, goose, and butter. Also, eat avocados and cook with olive oil. Fatty fish are a great way to get omega 3 fatty acids. Heavy cream, yogurt, and cheese can be consumed more than usual.

   * Drink black tea, black coffee, water, and bone broth. Don't add sugar to your beverages. Any dairy you consume should be full-fat and not a diet or

low-fat variant.

* Nuts are allowed, but they should be low in carbs. Have nuts like pecans and macadamia nuts that are high in fat.

Foods to Avoid on the Keto Diet

Here is a list of foods that you should not eat while on the keto diet:

* Cut off processed foods as much as possible. Wholesome natural foods are recommended. Get rid of your stock of candies, sugary cereals, sodas, cookies, etc. A lot of the "healthy" labeled processed foods contain hidden sugars, so avoid those too. Avoid artificial sweeteners like Equal as well.

* Avoid eating too many fruits because they have a lot of natural sugars. Moderate consumption of

berries is ok.

* Avoid any starchy foods. This includes starchy vegetables like potatoes. Also, avoid pasta and white rice. Lower your consumption of lentils and beans too.

* Avoid alcohol, especially beer. Wine is more keto-friendly but should be consumed in moderation.

* Avoid margarine, and don't try to substitute it for butter.

* Use these lists to guide you on your next grocery trip. Buy more keto-friendly foods and avoid buying anything that might cause you to compromise the state of ketosis you have been trying to induce.

More Benefits of the Keto Diet

- It allows you to eat until you are satisfied. You don't have to starve yourself or eat small portions to lose weight. The keto diet lets you eat until satiety, so you don't have to exercise control to stay on a diet. Try to avoid overeating if you aim to lose weight but have all of your main meals on time.

- It does not require calorie counting. Most fad diets or other weight-loss diets will require serious calorie counting. This means you have to ensure that you don't cross a particular threshold of calories per day or per meal. This can be a time consuming and limiting exercise. The keto diet allows you to eat freely without using any calorie calculators. The diet advocates against the consumption of foods that are even labeled low-calorie or no-calorie.

- It promotes better heart health. The modern-day diet has taken a toll on the body and can cause serious heart issues. Studies show that the keto diet promotes good heart health, despite the stigma against fats. Healthy fats will increase good cholesterol levels and lower bad cholesterol levels in your body. A high carb diet with trans fats and refined oils is what causes higher levels of bad LDL in your body. This causes blockage in arteries and can lead to heart diseases.

- It helps to increase energy levels and focus. While it might be the opposite during the initial keto-adaptation phase, you will notice that the keto diet enables you to be more focused and feel re-energized. A high carb diet can leave you feeling tired soon after the body breaks down the carbs. This will make you tired and hungry again. This diet will help you be more productive and be able to focus on your work all day long.

- It will also help in reducing unhealthy cravings.

A high carb diet with sugar will increase the incidence of untimely cravings. The body takes more time to burn fat, so you will be less likely to eat between meals. The high carb diet will make you feel hungry as soon as the body burns through the meal. Eating sugars and processed foods can cause an imbalance in hormones as well. This is countered by the keto diet.

- It can help in the regulation of triglyceride levels in your body. Low-fat consumption causes higher levels of triglycerides. Increasing fat consumption will allow the triglyceride level to come back to a normal level again.

- It can lower hypertension and the risk of it. A high carb diet causes an increase in blood pressure. This can then lead to the development of hypertension. Hypertension should be treated as soon as possible, because it can cause other health issues when it gets severe.

- It can help in treating irritable bowel syndrome. A diet that is high in carbs is likely to cause digestive problems and also irritable bowel syndrome. The keto diet can ease this problem and reduce the chances of any such condition.

- It helps reduce inflammation in the body. The keto diet can reduce inflammation caused by a high carbohydrate diet. This can help in pain management related to various inflammatory conditions.

- It helps to burn visceral fat, which is usually hard to get rid of. A high carb diet will result in the accumulation of fat in the abdominal region and cause belly fat. The keto diet can help in the reduction of this fat in an effective way.

There are many other benefits of the keto diet

that you will learn about if you try the diet yourself.

Why Do People Fail on Keto?

Now it's time to cut to the chase and talk about the mistakes many people make when keto-ing (real word, I promise!). The keto diet in and of itself should not be as challenging as some people make it out to be. Let's look at the mistakes, one by one.

1. *"Just a diet"*

The first mistake people make when keto-ing might seem obvious but is well worth looking at as a cause for failure. This is the perception they have of keto as 'just a diet' and they treat it as if it were in the same boat as fad diets or restrictive diets. It's not! When you approach keto as if it is just a diet, you'll end up seeing it as a chore, as some kind of difficult task to maintain in order to get anywhere. **This is such a big, yet common mistake.**

Of course, we can't deny that diets in general do involve changing eating habits (they don't *have* to though - see my book 'Keto Without Compromise' for more info) but with keto, you cannot come into the diet thinking that it's going to torture you and make you hungry 24/7. It's a lifestyle choice and if you aren't enjoying it, you're either doing it completely wrong or you shouldn't be looking to keto at all and it isn't the thing for you!

Conversely, you shouldn't approach keto thinking that EVERYTHING is allowed. Another big cause of failure with keto is when people who attempt it believe that keto allows you to non-keto now and then. It doesn't. When you reintroduce foods into your system that inevitably will prevent the healing process of ketosis and slow your weight loss progress, it's a dangerous and slippery slope. Sure, in theory, a candy bar every now and then will not affect you much, but the people who I've spoken to and mentored have not had this self-control. For many, one slip up becomes more regular than is anticipated. As humans, we have a remarkably low amount of will power and we have a talent for justifying bad habits. "Oh it's just a candy bar"… "Oh it's just two candy bars"… "Oh I'll try again next week with my diet."

The bottom line is this - take keto somewhat seriously but ensure you are fulfilled and enjoying the foods you are taking in. Don't see it as a diet and with a little effort, you'll end up taking on better habits that will lead to weight loss, a healthier body and a happier you (see the introduction for how keto helps with mood and self-esteem).

2. Accurate Calorie Count

This one is a big one! A huge one actually. A mistake that I would say 90% of all people who have ever dieted in any way make is that they misrepresent how many calories they eat and don't take into consideration that calories, even small amounts of them exist in drinks and snacks. These do add up!

A lot of people go on the keto diet and ask me why it's been three weeks and the pounds haven't dropped or their weight has even INCREASED! The mechanism behind this is simple - are you consciously aware of your daily calorie intake? The way the body works at a basic level for weight loss (not accounting for muscle loss etc) is that if you are eating less calories than your body burns, you lose weight. Keto speeds up the metabolism making this easier but won't help you to lose weight in every way. You need to be making an effort to ensure calories are not excessive. For example, olive oil is a big component of keto-ing and yet, while it is healthy, two large tablespoons comes to 198 calories! These contribute to daily intake so you need to be more rigid with your calorie awareness if you are not seeing results by week three. However, I AM NOT advocating for unhealthy eating habits where you obsess over calories. Just some awareness of the general habits you have concerning food goes a long way.

3. Results & Sticking It Out

Another major reason why people fail on keto is they don't stick it out for long enough and get discouraged when results don't come quickly enough. If you're one of these people, you need to take note of something. Ketosis takes varying amounts of time in everyone. No-one is the same so if you read somewhere that one person was able to fully restore and heal their body in a week and then they began shedding pounds like butter in a pan, don't compare this person's results to your own! I once met a lady who took 5 months for her body to restart and she eventually lost even more weight than the people who keto-ed a long time before her.

Stick it out and the results will come. Human biology is complex but simple at the same time. Overall, our bodily mechanisms function in more or less the same way.

4. Water

This reason for failure cannot be overstated. You need to drink a daily amount of 2 litres or else you will find weight loss and ketosis nearly impossible! We are 80% water and we require it for every cellular process in our bodies. Some studies suggest that nearly 3/4 of Americans are chronically dehydrated - that means 75% of us are living in a state of dehydration. Keto requires water, as do you! Drink, drink, drink and stay away from alcohol as much as you can!

The Keto Kitchen

Before we go any further, it's time to stock up. The success to keto comes with what you buy, what your kitchen looks like and what you put into your body. This chapter addresses the first of these two concerns.

You need a range of ingredients which will become the staple of your fridge, cupboards and diet. Knowing what to buy when at the supermarket leaves out the guesswork and prevents you from being tempted into old habits. So stay away from the candy and confectionary and make note of the following must-have ingredients for a Keto diet.

1.Filling, Low Carbohydrate, Non-Starchy Vegetables

We're going to dig deeper here, don't worry - I'm not just pointing out the obvious. When you include low carb veggies into your daily diet, you'll notice a change in the way your body works. Immediately, you'll notice how filling these vegetables are and how your portion size reduces quite rapidly. For the first two or three days, you might feel lethargic if you aren't used to incorporating vegetables into your daily eating habits. Stick with it though! Your body is processing these goodies and very soon, you'll learn to love them and so will your body. You'll feel the effects after a week: no headaches, grogginess or generalized fatigue.

You might also notice that your bowl movements become more frequent. This is because non-starchy low-carb vegetables are antioxidants. They act as detoxifiers for your gut and immune system. So, which vegetables should you be putting into your shopping basket? **Ones that are high in vitamin C, K, and D**. Here are some suggestions but you don't need to be adding all of them. Try some and see which ones you like. It's so important when keto-ing that you enjoy everything you eat. We're in this for the long haul, am I right?

Vegetables:

- Kale
- Spinach
- Broccoli
- Cauliflower
- Brussel Sprouts
- Zucchini (*Courgette* for readers of the EU, the UK, NZ and AUS)
- Carrots

Remember that these vegetables are also formidable sources of dietary fibre and so play a pivotal role in keeping your digestive system healthy and in check. Fibre prevents constipation, irritable bowel syndrome and problems of indigestion.

2. Fish

Now, remember that while we are maintaining a low-carb diet, moderate to high protein is essential too. Proteins help to maintain brain health, muscle health, replenish and rejuvenate cells and keep the organism healthy. Fish and seafood is the perfect source for keto dieters because unlike red meat, we don't get the backlash of bad fats and high iron concentration. A lot of fish is also high in B vitamins, omega 3, potassium and between you and me - it's basically carb free! If you aren't a fan of fish or seafood, you needn't worry just move on to number 3 but for those willing to give it a go, here are some must-try fish based ingredients for the keto diet.

- Salmon

- Squid

- Tuna (be careful with tuna since it can be high in mercury!)

- Shellfish such as mussels

3. Avocados

Okay let's be honest - you saw this one coming. It wouldn't be a keto cookbook without me shoving AVOCADOS into every free line of the page, right? Well while these wholesome fruits have a bad reputation in the media and are associated with the millennial student diet, there is a reason so many people are picking them up these days. They're awfully popular and with good reason too! In fact, I'd go as far as saying they are essential for the keto diet and it's almost impossible to find keto success without them. Why?

1. Very low in carbs (9g per 100g of fruit)

2. High potassium

3. Low cholesterol

4. Loaded with fibre

5. 26% of daily Vitamin K

6. 18-20% of daily Vitamin C

7. Source of Vitamins E, B6 and B5

8. Low in calories

9. 0 sodium - good for lowering blood pressure

Need I say more?

--

4. Lean Chicken

In the past, I've advised people to pick up chicken when keto-ing but unfortunately, they don't pay attention to what kind of chicken they are buying and eating. Lean cuts of chicken and ones that aren't lean could not be further removed. It's like apples and oranges in terms of difference. In essence, you want to be free range corn-fed chicken fillets. That's a mouthful to say but ideally that's the cut you want to buy and in my experience living in both the United States and in the United Kingdom, these are pretty much available at any supermarket and/or butcher. If worse comes to worst, regular chicken fillets will do. As long as you aren't buying pre-cooked or fried chicken, you're one step ahead of the game as far as the keto diet is concerned.

5. Olive Oil

You want to know why the Greeks and general population of the Mediterranean have such great skin, flowing shiny hair and look great for their age? Well the answer is olive oil. They use it in everything. From Morocco to Italy, it's used in every dish and you need to be replacing any form of butter and oil in your house with olive oil. Why? Because olive oil isn't really an oil at all. It's rich in mono-fats, prevents heart disease, cancer, strokes and liver disease. It also possesses hydrating and replenishing qualities for the hair, nails and skin. Yes, this oil is more expensive but at this point, your best bet is to buy a big bottle of 'extra virgin' olive oil and use small amounts in everything you make. Whether it's a salad or you're frying an egg, anything you would use oil or butter for, olive oil is your super hero. It literally is the fountain of youth we kept hearing about in old movies.

6. Nuts and Seeds

High in protein and unsaturated fat, these are your go-to snack from now on. If you have to transition into them by buying coated or salted, fine. However, do try to eat them 'nude'.

Nuts to Try:

- Cashews

- Walnuts

- Chia seeds

- Flaxseeds

- Sesame seeds

- Brazil nuts

You probably noticed that 'peanuts' are not on the list. Sorry, but their health benefits are minimal and they're a food you should save for a treat and should not be eaten as a staple of a quotidian healthy diet.

7. Fruit

Very few food items can be eaten in such copious amounts but I will say sparingly that you can eat pretty much as much fruit as you'd like. However, there are some fruits which are better for keto diets than others. These include:

1. Blackberries
2. Strawberries
3. Blueberries
4. Cranberries
5. Oranges
6. Red apples
7. Bananas

8. Dark Chocolate

There has to be a silver lining somewhere right? Well there is! All I ask is that you replace your current chocolate habits with dark chocolate (preferably a chocolate that has a high Cocoa percentage - upwards of 60%). Dark chocolate is good for heart health, blood pressure and reducing stress.

9. Brown Rice and Brown Pasta

Similar to other carbs, we need to keep this on the down-low but you need *some* carbs for a healthy diet. Substitute any carb you'd normally have with the brown alternative. The same applies to breads - opt for wholegrain instead of white.

10. Eggs

A cheap, healthy and easily accessible form of protein which is high in B vitamins and low in calories. You can use eggs instead of other proteins which makes them versatile. Duck, goose or chicken eggs will do.

- -

Needless to say, the rest is down to you as you craft your keto diet. Make sure whatever other foods you pick up, that they're keto-friendly - low carb, moderate protein, high fat. Nonetheless, these ten items should be your go to whenever you enter a store to do your weekly grocery shopping.

Now it's time to get to cooking.

Keto Recipe Cookbook

Now that you have all the introductory information you need to keto success, it's time to dive into some meals (breakfast, lunch and dinner) and how to prepare them. This is called 'meal prep'. Meal prep is a question of efficiency, cost and speed. Nobody wants to be spending absurd amounts of money or time preparing their meals. Even those who love cooking do not want the hassle of ridiculous investment in kitchen items, exotic individual ingredients and so on.

In the next three chapters, cost-efficient and delicious meals have been laid out in a way that is easy to navigate - with ingredients, specific cooking times, directions and serving sizes, keto meal prep will be easier than ever...

Breakfast Meal Prep

Keto Cereal

Serves: 3

Ingredients:

- 1 1/2 cup of almonds

- 2 tablespoons of flax and chia seeds

- 1 teaspoon of vanilla extract

- 1 pinch of salt

- 1 medium egg

- 1/2 cup of coconut oil

- 1 cup coconut flakes

- 1 teaspoon of clove

- 1/2 tablespoon cinnamon

- 1 cup of walnuts

- 1/2 cup of sesame seeds

Directions:

- In a bowl, mix the flakes, seeds and nuts together and stir the vanilla in with the cinnamon, cloves, and salt.

- Heat oven to 320°.

- Stir and beat egg and mix with the other ingredients in bowl. Mix everything together.

- Place mix on a baking tray and bake entire dish for 30 minutes.

- When cooked, let it cool for ten minutes.

- Serve in bowl with milk or yoghurt of choice.

Keto Eggs

Serves: 8

Ingredients:

4 teaspoons butter

2 Roma tomatoes, chopped

8 eggs

Pepper to taste

Salt to taste

4 teaspoons olive oil

4 green onions, thinly sliced; keep the white and green parts separate

4 tablespoons milk

Directions:

- Place a skillet over medium heat. Add oil and butter. When butter melts, add the whites of the green onion and sauté until translucent.

- Add tomatoes and green part of the green onions and cook until slightly dry.

- Meanwhile, add milk and eggs in a bowl and whisk them well.

- Pour eggs into the pan and stir constantly until the eggs are cooked.

- Season with salt and pepper and serve.

Keto-Style Hash Browns

Serves: 2

Ingredients:

3 medium eggs

1/2 teaspoon of garlic powder

Pinch of salt

Pinch of White Pepper

1 cup of peeled/shredded cabbage

1/2 sliced onion

1 tablespoon of olive oil

Directions:

- In a bowl, mix eggs, pepper, salt and garlic together.

- Now mix the onion, cabbage and eggs.

- Heat a frying pan and add the oil. At this stage, you need to divide the mix into patties and shape them accordingly.

- Fry until cooked, usually 4 minutes on each side.

Eggy Brekky Cups

Serves: 6

Ingredients:

1 1/2 pounds of minced beef

1 tablespoon of rosemary

2 cloves of garlic

1 teaspoon of cumin

1/2 teaspoon of black pepper

1 teaspoon of salt

1 cup of spinach

1 cup of cheese of choice (cheddar is recommended)

6 medium eggs

1 tablespoon of chives

Directions:

- Preheat oven to 380°.

- Mix beef, herbs and spices in a bowl.

- Using cupcake tins, place a handful of meat and fill them.

- Garnish each with the cheddar and spinach, accordingly.

- Crack the eggs over each tin and bake until the meat is cooked. This should take half an hour.

- When cooked, let it cool and garnish with the remaining chives.

Sausage Breakfast Sandwich

Serves: 2

Ingredients:

2 large eggs

4 sausage patties

4 tablespoons sharp cheddar cheese

1 teaspoon sriracha sauce or to taste

¼ teaspoon red pepper flakes (optional)

2 tablespoons cream cheese

Little butter, grease

Directions:

- Whisk together eggs, red pepper flakes, salt and pepper in a bowl.

- Add cream cheese and sharp cheddar cheese into a microwave-safe bowl. Cook for 20 seconds or until it melts. Add sriracha sauce and stir.

- Place a skillet over medium flame. Add a little butter and let it melt.

- Pour ½ the beaten egg mixture. Spread half the cheese mixture in the center of the omelet and let it cook for a minute.

- Fold the edges of the omelet over the cheese. Carefully slide on to a plate.

- Repeat steps 3-5 and make the remaining omelet.

Meanwhile, heat the patties following the instructions on the package.

- Place 2 patties on a serving platter. Place one omelet on each patty. Place the remaining 2 patties over the omelet to complete the sandwiches.

Blueberry Cupcakes (Keto-Style)

Serves: 6

Ingredients:

1 cup of flour

1/5 of a cup of brown sugar

1 pinch of salt

1/3 teaspoon of baking soda

1/4 cup of soya milk (cashew/almond milk can be used)

1/3 teaspoon of baking powder

1/4 cup of melted butter

2 medium/large eggs

1/2 teaspoon of vanilla extract

1/2 cup of blueberries (frozen or fresh)

Directions:

- In a bowl, combine the flour with the baking soda, powder, and salt. Now, add in milk, the eggs and vanilla. Whisk well.

- Add blueberries ensuring they do not get squashed. Folding works best under layers of the batter.

- Use a spoon to evenly scoop the batter into muffin or cupcake liners.

- Bake for 20 to 30 minutes.

- Allow cupcakes to cool and then serve.

Spanish Baked Eggs

Serves: 4

Ingredients:

2 tablespoons olive oil

1 teaspoon paprika

2 tomatoes, sliced

Salt to taste

Pepper to taste

4 ounces manchego cheese, grated

2 chorizo sausages, chopped

½ teaspoon ground cumin

2/3 cup roasted peppers strips

4 eggs

2 teaspoons finely chopped parsley

Directions:

- Place a pan on medium flame and heat some oil. When the oil is heated, add chorizo, cumin, and paprika and cook for 4-5 minutes until cooked thoroughly.

- Add tomatoes and cook until the tomatoes are mashed. Stir in the roasted pepper, pepper and salt and mix well. Turn off the heat.

- Take 4 small baking dishes. Divide the mixture equally into the dishes. Spread it all over the dishes. Make a cavity in the center of each dish, big enough for an egg to fit in.

- Break an egg into each cavity. Scatter cheese and parsley on top.

- Bake in a preheated oven at 390° F for about 5-10 minutes, depending on the desired doneness.

- Serve hot.

Keto Bell Eggs

Serves: 3

Ingredients:

1 Bell Pepper

4 large eggs (or 5 medium eggs)

1/2 teaspoon of salt

1 teaspoon of black pepper

1 tablespoon of parsley (chopped)

1 tablespoon of olive oil

1/2 an avocado

Directions:

- Start by heating the olive oil over a medium-high heat in a frying pan.

- Chop the bell pepper into ring shapes and fry for three minutes each. One and a half minutes on each side.

- Next, crack an egg into each pepper ensuring
there is no overspill. The eggs should be cooked to
your liking but an average of two minutes is
recommended.

- Add the salt and pepper to the yolk of the eggs.

- Once served on plate, use the parsley for
garnishing.

- The avocado can be served on the side or
smashed to be eaten as a high-fat, healthy dip.

Cheddar Cheese and Bacon Balls

Serves: 14-16 (3-4 balls per serving)

Ingredients:

10-11 ounces bacon

10-11 ounces cheddar cheese

10-11 ounces cream cheese

4 ounces butter, at room temperature, divided

1 teaspoon chili flakes (optional)

1 teaspoon pepper (optional)

Salt to taste

Directions:

Place a pan over medium heat. Add half the butter and melt. Add bacon and cook until crisp. Remove bacon with a slotted spoon and place on paper towels.

When cool enough to handle, crumble the bacon. Set aside in a shallow bowl.

Pour the remaining fat from the pan into a bowl. Add remaining butter, cheddar cheese, cream cheese, chili flakes, pepper and salt and mix well, using your hands.

Chill for 20-30 minutes.

Divide the mixture into 40-50 portions and shape into balls.

Dredge the mixture in bacon and serve.

Store leftovers in an airtight container in the refrigerator.

Black and White Fat Bombs

Serves: 24

Ingredients:

4 cups slivered almonds

3-4 tablespoons swerve or erythritol

2 teaspoons grated orange zest

4 tablespoons unsweetened cocoa powder

2 cups virgin or extra-virgin coconut oil

4 teaspoons vanilla extract

¼ teaspoon kosher salt

Directions:

- Take 2 mini muffin tins of 12 counts each. Place disposable liners in it.

- Add almonds, swerve, orange zest, oil, vanilla and salt into the food processor. Process until smooth.

- Divide equally into 2 bowls. Add cocoa powder into one of the bowls and mix well.

- Spoon vanilla mixture in one half of the muffin cup and immediately fill the remaining half portion with cocoa mixture. Tap the muffin tin on your countertop lightly for the mixture to settle.

- Place in the freezer until firm. Remove from the freezer and remove from the muffin tin.

- Transfer into an airtight container and refrigerate until use. It can last for 5 days.

Fudgy Macadamia Chocolate Fat Bombs

Serves: 12

Ingredients:

4 ounces cocoa butter

4 tablespoons swerve

½ cup heavy cream or coconut oil

4 tablespoons cocoa powder, unsweetened

8 ounces macadamia nuts, chopped

Directions:

- Add cocoa butter into a heatproof bowl. Place the bowl in a double boiler until the cocoa butter melts. Stir occasionally. Remove the bowl from the double boiler.

- Add cocoa powder and swerve and mix well.

- Add macadamia nuts and mix well. Divide the mixture into 12 fat bomb molds or paper candy cups. Cool completely.

- Refrigerate until firm.

- Remove from the refrigerator about 30 minutes before serving.

Creamsicle Fat Bombs

Serves: 20

Ingredients:

1 cup coconut oil

8 ounces cream cheese

20 drops liquid stevia or to taste

1 cup heavy whipping cream

2 teaspoons orange vanilla mio

Directions:

-Add coconut oil, cream cheese, stevia, whipping cream and orange vanilla mio into a bowl. Blend until smooth using an immersion blender. Just in case the ingredients are not blending well, then microwave on high for 20 seconds to soften.

- Pour into silicone tray or fat bomb molds.

- Freeze for a couple of hours or until firm.

- Remove from the mold and serve. Store the remaining fat bombs in an airtight container. This can be refrigerated until further use.

Cheesy Ham and Keto Eggs

Serves: 12

Ingredients:

2 tablespoons of olive oil (extra virgin preferable)

Ham slices (12 - one per serving)

1 teaspoon of salt

1 teaspoon of white pepper

Eggs (12 - one per serving)

1 cup of cheese (shredded cheddar preferable)

Directions:

- Start by turning oven on and preheating it to between 300 and 400°. Using the olive oil, grease 12 cupcake tins.

- Place the slices of ham in each as a base.

- This is followed by a sprinkling of cheese on top.

- Next, crack the eggs - one into each tin over the ham and cheese. Season each tin accordingly.

- Let the cups bake for between 10 and 20 minutes depending on how you like your eggs.

Lunch Meal Prep

Keto Meat Stack

Serves: 3

Ingredients:

1/2 pound of pork mince (or ground beef)

1 whole pressed avocado

1/2 teaspoon of salt

1/2 teaspoon of pepper

4 medium eggs

1 tablespoon of olive oil

Directions:

- Use the mince/ground meat and press it to form three patties.

- Next, heat the olive oil in a medium heat frying

pan.

- After, cook the patties for four minutes on each side. Once cooked, spread the mashed avocado onto the patties.

- Keeping the pan hot, fry the eggs and place on top of the avocado.

- Serve.

Neapolitan Parmesan Eggs

Serves: 4

Ingredients:

1 cup of parmesan (grated)

4 slices of ham (chopped)

1/2 teaspoon of salt

1/2 teaspoon of pepper

1 teaspoon of chilli flakes

Directions:

- Preheat your oven to 380° and use olive oil to grease a baking tray.

- Prepare two bowls. You now need to crack the eggs ensuring the whites go in one and the yolks in another.

- Beat the egg whites until thickening begins to

occur (usually after 2-4 minutes).

- Add cheese and ham followed by salt and pepper seasoning.

- Using a spoon, add six to eight dollops of egg whites to the tray and burrow in the centre to make space.

- Bake for five minutes.

- Next, using the spoon, add the egg yolk to the centre of the whites.

- Season accordingly with chilli flakes and bake for another five minutes.

- Serve.

Keto Chicken Soup

Serves: 4

Ingredients:

2 medium cauliflowers, cut into florets

2 cups chicken broth

1 teaspoon sea salt

Freshly ground pepper to taste

¼ teaspoon dried thyme

½ cup cooked, finely chopped chicken thighs

1 1/3 cups almond milk, unsweetened

2 teaspoons onion powder

½ teaspoon garlic powder

¼ teaspoon celery seeds (optional)

½ cup Collagen protein beef gelatin (optional)

Directions:

- Add cauliflower, broth, salt, pepper, thyme, milk, onion powder, garlic powder and celery seeds into a soup pot.

- Place the soup pot over medium heat. Cover with a lid.

- When it boils, lower heat and simmer until cauliflower is soft.

- Turn off the heat. Take out about a cup of the cooked liquid and add into a bowl.

- Add a teaspoon of gelatin at a time into the bowl of cooked liquid. Whisk well each time until the gelatin is dissolved. Continue doing this until the entire gelatin is added.

- Pour the gelatin mixture into a blender. Also add the cooked cauliflower mixture.

- Blend until smooth and creamy.

- Pour the soup back into the pot. Place the pot over low heat.

- Add chicken and stir. Cover and heat thorough-ly.

- Ladle into soup bowls and serve.

Asparagus & Sorrel Bisque

Serves: 4

Ingredients:

1 tablespoon unsalted butter

1 large leek, thinly sliced

½ teaspoon kosher salt or to taste

Pepper to taste

1 pound asparagus, trimmed

¼ cup crème Fraiche

1 tablespoon extra-virgin olive oil

1 stalk green garlic, sliced

2 cups low sodium vegetable broth

2 cups sorrel or baby arugula + extra to garnish

1 radish, sliced, to garnish

Directions:

- Place a soup pot over medium heat. Add oil and butter. When butter melts, add leeks, green garlic and asparagus and stir for a minute.

- Add salt, pepper and broth.

- Cover and cook until asparagus is tender. Turn off the heat.

- Cool completely.

- Pour soup into a bowl and keep in the refrigerator for 2-3 hours. Do not cover the bowl.

- Remove the chilled soup from the refrigerator and transfer into a blender.

- Add sorrel and blend for 40 to 50 seconds or

until smooth.

- Taste and adjust the seasoning if required.

- Ladle into soup bowls. Sprinkle some pepper on top. Top with a tablespoon of crème Fraiche in each bowl.

- Place radish slices on top and serve.

Avocado Cucumber Gazpacho

Serves: 3

Ingredients:

1 medium cucumber, peeled, deseeded, chopped

½ jalapeño, deseeded, chopped

1 medium avocado, peeled, pitted, chopped

2 tablespoons apple cider vinegar

½ teaspoon salt or to taste

Pepper to taste

A handful fresh cilantro or basil, chopped

1 clove garlic, peeled, chopped

Directions:

- Add cucumber, jalapeño, avocado, cilantro, vinegar, salt, pepper and garlic into a blender and blend for 30-40 seconds.

- Add water and blend until smooth.

- Taste and adjust the seasoning if required.

- Pour into a bowl. Cover and refrigerate until use.

- Ladle into soup bowls and serve.

Ultimate Keto Egg Salad

Serves: 3-4

Ingredients:

5 rashers of bacon

4 tablespoons of red wine vinegar

1 teaspoon of mustard

1/2 teaspoon of salt

1/2 teaspoon of pepper

5 tablespoons of olive oil

3 medium eggs

4-5 cups of spinach

1/2 cup of feta cheese

handful of cherry tomatoes

Directions:

- In a frying pan, fry the bacon and allow fats to
sweat with a tablespoon of olive oil. Fry until very

crispy.

- Once cooked, place bacon aside on a plate and let it rest. When room temperature or safe to handle, half of the bacon needs to be crumbled into small pieces and the other half should be cut up into small slices.

- Now, it's time to make the dressing for the salad. Mix the vinegar with the mustard and seasonings in a bowl. Whisk in the rest of the olive oil. Add the bacon crumblings.

- Fry the eggs in the pan.

- In a bowl, mix the tomatoes, spinach, feta, remaining bacon pieces and add the dressing.

- The salad needs to be portioned with the eggs on top. Serve.

Coleslaw-Stuffed Wraps

Serves: 2 (4 wraps each)

Ingredients:

For the coleslaw:

1 ½ cups red cabbage, thinly sliced

6 tablespoons keto-friendly mayonnaise

A pinch salt or to taste

1 green onion, chopped

1 teaspoon apple cider vinegar

Other ingredients:

8 collard leaves, discard stems

3 tablespoons packed alfalfa sprouts

½ pound ground meat of your choice, cooked, chilled

Directions:

- To make coleslaw: Add cabbage, mayonnaise,

salt, green onion and vinegar into a bowl and mix well.

- To make wraps: Place collard leaves on your countertop.

- Place a spoonful of the coleslaw on the edge of each of the leaves, opposite the stem part.

- Tuck the sides and roll the leaves. Fasten with toothpicks.

- Serve.

Cuban Keto 'Get Up and Go' Salad

Serves: 3

Ingredients:

3 chayote's, peeled

Salt to taste

Pepper to taste

¼ teaspoon mustard powder

2 tablespoons extra-virgin olive oil

Directions:

- Place a pot filled with water and chayote over medium heat.

- Cook until tender. Drain off the water.

- Cool for a while. Chop into 1-inch cubes.

- Add oil, salt, pepper and mustard into a bowl.

- Whisk well and pour over the chayote.

- Toss well. Refrigerate for at least an hour.

- Serve as it is or over lettuce leaves.

Cobb Salad with Ranch Dressing

Serves: 4

Ingredients:

4 eggs, hardboiled, peeled, chopped

1 rotisserie chicken, chopped

2 avocados, peeled, pitted, chopped

2 tablespoons chopped chives

6 ounces bacon

4 ounces blue cheese

2 tomatoes, chopped

10 ounces iceberg lettuce

Salt to taste

Pepper to taste

For ranch dressing:

6 tablespoons keto-friendly mayonnaise

4 tablespoons water

2 tablespoons ranch seasoning

Salt to taste

Directions:

- For the dressing: Toss all the dressing ingredients in a bowl and mix well. Keep it aside so that the flavors can come out.

- Place a pan over medium flame. Add bacon and cook until it becomes crisp. Remove and place on a plate.

- When cool enough to handle, crumble the bacon. Set aside.

- To assemble: Spread lettuce leaves on a serving platter. Scatter the rest of the ingredients of salad over the lettuce.

- Pour dressing on top. Sprinkle chives and bacon on top and serve.

Blueberry Salad

Serves: 2-3

Ingredients:

20 blueberries or any other berries of your choice

2 large bags salad leaves

4 teaspoons lemon juice

4 tablespoons coconut oil

1 small onion, sliced

4 tablespoons olive oil

2 large chicken breasts, chopped

Salt to taste

Pepper to taste

Directions:

- Place a pan over medium flame. Add coconut oil. When cool enough to handle, add chicken, salt and pepper and cook until tender. Turn off the heat and cool completely.

- Transfer into a serving bowl. Add onion, blueberries, lemon juice, salad leaves and oil and toss
well.

- Serve.

Keto Hot Chicken Salad

Serves: 2

Ingredients:

1 boneless chicken breast half, halved lengthwise

Himalayan pink salt to taste

½ avocado, peeled, pitted, chopped

1 medium tomato, chopped

¼ red onion, chopped

10 basil leaves, chopped

½ tablespoon olive oil

Pepper to taste

1.8 ounces mozzarella balls

½ jar artichoke hearts

3 stalks asparagus, trimmed, chopped into 2-3 inch pieces

2 cups baby spinach

For dressing:

1 tablespoon extra-virgin olive oil

½ teaspoon Dijon mustard

Himalayan pink salt to taste

¾ teaspoon balsamic vinegar

1 small clove garlic, peeled, minced

Pepper to taste

Directions:

- Season the chicken with salt and pepper.

- Place a cast iron skillet over medium flame. Heat some oil and add chicken and cook for 3 minutes or until it becomes golden brown. Flip and cook both sides until it turns golden brown and is cooked through.

- Place asparagus next to the chicken and cook until the asparagus gets soft. Turn off the heat.

- To make dressing: Add all the ingredients of dressing into a small jar. Fasten the lid and shake the jar vigorously until well combined. Set aside for about 30 mins for the flavors to set in.

- To serve: Place spinach on a serving platter. Top with chicken, artichoke, avocado, onion, mozzarella and basil.

- Drizzle dressing on top and serve.

Cucumber Salad

Serves: 4

Ingredients:

1 pound cucumbers, quartered lengthwise and then sliced

4 tablespoons lemon juice

4 tablespoons mayonnaise

Freshly ground pepper to taste

Salt to taste

Directions:

- Add lemon juice, mayonnaise, salt and pepper into a bowl and stir.

- Add cucumber and stir until well coated with the dressing.

Tuna Fish Salad

Serves: 2

Ingredients:

4 cups mixed greens

½ cup chopped fresh parsley leaves

20 large kalamata olives, pitted

1 avocado, peeled, pitted, diced

2 cans light tuna in water, drained, chopped

2 large tomatoes, diced

½ cup chopped fresh mint leaves,

2 small zucchini, sliced lengthwise

2 green onions, sliced

2 tablespoons extra-virgin olive oil

½ teaspoon Himalayan sea salt or fine sea salt

2 tablespoons balsamic vinegar

Freshly cracked pepper to taste

Directions:

- Preheat a cast iron skillet or grill pan. Place zucchini slices on it and grill on both sides. Remove the grilled zucchini and place on your cutting board.

- When it's cool enough, chop into bite-sized pieces.

- Add zucchini into a large bowl. Add mixed greens, parsley leaves, kalamata olives, avocado, tuna, tomatoes, mint leaves, zucchini, green onions, extra-virgin olive oil, salt, balsamic vinegar and cracked pepper.

- Toss well.

- Serve right away.

Turkey-Cheddar Roll-Ups

Serves: 2

Ingredients:

6 slices deli turkey

6 slices cheese

Avocado slices

Cucumber slices

Blueberries

Chopped almonds

Directions:

Place turkey slices on a serving platter. Place a slice of cheese on each.

Place avocado, cucumber, blueberries and almonds. Roll the turkey slices and place with the seam side facing down.

Tofu Frittata

Serves: 4-8

Ingredients:

2 tablespoons olive oil

2 zucchinis, chopped

2 packages firm or extra firm tofu

1 cup nondairy milk of your choice

1 teaspoon dried basil

1 teaspoon ground cumin

½ teaspoon red pepper flakes

4 scallions, chopped

1 large red onion, chopped

15-16 crimini mushrooms, chopped

6 tablespoons nutritional yeast

2 tablespoons arrowroot

½ teaspoon turmeric

Salt to taste
Pepper to taste

2 tomatoes, chopped

½ cup chopped kalamata olives

Cooking spray

Directions:

Grease a casserole dish with cooking spray.

Place a large skillet over medium heat. Add oil and heat. Add onion and sauté until translucent.

Stir in zucchini and mushrooms and sauté until tender. Add salt and pepper to taste and stir. Turn off the heat.

Add tofu, nutritional yeast, milk, arrowroot, cumin, turmeric, basil, salt, pepper and red pepper flakes into a blender and blend until creamy.

Pour over the zucchini mixture and stir.

Transfer into the prepared casserole dish.

Scatter tomatoes, olives and scallions on top.

Bake in a preheated oven at 375 ° F for 45-60 minutes or until frittata is set and top is golden brown.

Remove from the oven and cool for a few minutes.

Cut into wedges and serve.

Zucchini Crust Grilled

Serves: 4

Ingredients:

For zucchini crust bread slices:

8 cups shredded zucchini

1 cup shredded mozzarella cheese

2 teaspoons dried oregano

Pepper to taste

2 eggs

½ cup grated parmesan cheese

Salt to taste

For cheese:

2/3 cup grated sharp cheddar cheese

2 tablespoons butter, at room temperature

Directions:

Place rack in the center of the oven. Place a sheet of parchment paper on a baking sheet. Spray some cooking spray over it.

Add zucchini into a microwave safe bowl and cook on high for 6 minutes.

Place the zucchini on a dishcloth. Bring the ends of the dishcloth together and squeeze the zucchini of excess moisture. Squeeze as much as possible.

Add zucchini, mozzarella cheese, egg, Parmesan cheese, oregano and seasoning. Mix well.

Make 8 equal portions of the mixture and place on the prepared baking sheet.

Form squares of the mixture.

Bake in a preheated oven at 375 ° F for 20 minutes or until light golden brown.

Take out the baking sheet from the oven and let the zucchini bread cool completely.

Carefully remove the zucchini bread crust from the parchment paper.

To assemble: Spread butter on one side of the zucchini bread.

Place a nonstick skillet over medium heat. Place zucchini bread on the skillet, with the buttered side facing down.

Sprinkle about 3 tablespoons cheese over it. Cover with another zucchini bread, butter side facing up. Cook until the underside is golden brown.

Flip sides and cook the other side until golden brown.

Repeat steps 10-13 and make the remaining sandwiches.

Spinach Artichoke Chicken Casserole

Serves: 12

Ingredients:

20 ounces artichoke hearts

8 ounces full fat cream cheese

2 cups parmesan cheese, divided

6 cloves garlic, peeled, minced

20 ounces frozen, chopped spinach, drained, squeezed of excess moisture

8 ounces, full fat, keto-friendly mayonnaise

2 cups shredded mozzarella cheese, divided

2 bags chicken tenderloins, thawed, chopped into chunks

Directions:

Place chicken in a large baking dish. Sprinkle salt and pepper over it.

Bake in a preheated oven at 400°F for 15 minutes.

Meanwhile, add spinach, garlic, artichoke, half the cheeses, mayonnaise and cream cheese into a bowl and mix until well combined.

Remove the baking dish from the oven and spread the spinach mixture over the chicken.

Lower temperature to 350°F and bake for another 20 minutes.

Take the baking dish out of the oven and sprinkle the remaining Parmesan cheese and mozzarella cheese on top.

Set the oven to broil mode. Broil for a few minutes until cheese melts.

Serve.

Chicken Club Stuffed Avocados

Serves: 2

Ingredients:

3 ounces grilled, chicken, diced

1 avocado, halved, pitted

2 slices cooked bacon, crumbled

Juice of ½ lime

2 tablespoons mayonnaise

Salt to taste

Pepper to taste

1 small tomato, diced

A handful cilantro, chopped

Directions:

Carefully scoop the avocado but retain the avocado cases.

Add the scooped avocado into a bowl and mash it with a fork.

Add chicken, most of the bacon, 1-tablespoon lime juice, tomato, mayonnaise, half the cilantro, salt and pepper and mix well.

Fill this mixture in the retained avocado cases. Sprinkle remaining bacon and cilantro. Drizzle remaining lime juice on top and serve.

Iceburgers

Serves: 8

Ingredients:

2 large heads iceberg lettuce

2 red onions, cut into round slices

Salt to taste

8 slices cheddar cheese

Ranch dressing, to serve

8 slices bacon

2 pounds ground beef

Freshly ground pepper to taste

2 tomatoes, sliced

Directions:

Cut 16 large rounds from the iceberg lettuce. These are your buns.

Place a large skillet over medium flame. Add bacon and cook until crisp. Remove bacon with a slotted spoon and place on a plate lined with paper towels. Do not discard the fat in the pan.

Place onion slices and cook for 3 minutes. Flip sides and cook for 3 minutes. Remove onions and place on a plate. Discard the fat remaining in the pan.

Make 8 portions of the ground beef and shape into patties. Sprinkle salt and pepper on the burgers and place on the pan. Cook in batches if required.

Cook until the underside is brown. Flip sides and cook the other side until browned and cooked to the desired doneness.

Place a slice of cheese on each burger. Cover the pan for a few minutes so that the cheese melts.

Place one burger on each of 8 iceberg rounds. Place a slice of bacon on each. Place a tomato slice on each. Spoon some ranch dressing.

Cover with the remaining iceberg rounds. Fasten with toothpicks and serve.

Keto Quiche

Serves: 3

Ingredients:

1 ½ tablespoons coconut oil

1 medium bell peppers, chopped

2 cups chopped spinach

6 medium eggs, whisked

2 tablespoons chopped fresh basil

Salt to taste

Pepper to taste

3 slices bacon, diced

1 small onion, diced

1 small tomato, chopped

7-8 olives, sliced

2 cloves garlic, finely chopped

Salt to taste

Pepper to taste

6 tablespoons coconut cream

Directions:

Place a skillet over medium-high flame. Add oil and once it is heated, add bacon and cook until crisp. Take out the bacon and place on a plate lined with paper towels.

Add bell pepper and onion into the same pan and cook until tender.

Stir in the spinach and cook until spinach wilts. Turn off the heat and cool for 15 minutes.

Meanwhile, add eggs into a bowl and beat it well. Add tomatoes, olives, garlic, bacon, basil, coconut cream and spinach mixture. Mix well. Add salt and pepper to taste.

Pour into a baking dish.

Bake in a preheated oven at 350°F for 15 -30 minutes depending on how you like the eggs to be cooked.

Remove from the oven and allow it to cool for a few minutes.

Cut into 3 equal wedges and serve.

Dinner Meal Prep

Chicken Enchilada Bowl

Serves: 4

Ingredients:

1 tablespoon coconut oil

6 tablespoons keto-friendly red enchilada sauce

1 small onion, chopped

½ pound skinless, boneless chicken thighs

2 tablespoons water

½ can (from a 4 ounces can) diced green chilies

Toppings:

½ avocado, peeled, pitted, cubed

2 tablespoons chopped pickled jalapeños

1 small tomato, chopped

½ shredded cheese

4 tablespoons sour cream

To serve:

Cauliflower rice

Any other toppings of your choice

Directions:

- Place a skillet over medium heat. Add oil. When the oil is heated, add chicken and cook until light brown all over.

- Add enchilada sauce, onion, water and green chilies. Mix well.

- Lower the heat and cover with a lid. Simmer until chicken is cooked through.

- Remove chicken with a slotted spoon and place on your cutting board. When cool enough to handle, chop the chicken.

- Add chicken into the skillet. Simmer until thick.

- To assemble: Place cauliflower rice in 4 serving bowls.

- Divide the chicken among the bowls. Divide the avocado, jalapeño, tomato, cheese and sour cream among the bowls and serve.

Keto Meatball Feast

Serves: 4

Ingredients:

1 1/2 pounds of ground meat (pork/beef)

1 cup of cheddar

3 cloves of shredded garlic

1/2 cup of parmesan (grated)

2 medium eggs

3 tablespoons of olive oil

1 teaspoon of salt

1 onion

1 can of smashed or crushed tomatoes

2 teaspoons of pepper

2 teaspoons of oregano

Directions:

- Mix the beef, cheddar, 1 clove of garlic, parmesan and eggs in a bowl. Then add the salt. You may also add pepper or any other seasoning of your choice.

- With the mixture, form 12-14 small meatballs.

- In a frying pan, heat the olive oil.

- Cook the meatballs and turn regularly until all sides are gold. This takes between 8 and 12 minutes.

- Once cooked, set the meatballs aside.

- In the same pan, cook the onion until it is softened which takes 4 to 5 minutes.

- Mix the rest of the garlic in and cook for two minutes.

- Now, add the oregano, tomatoes and pepper.

- At this point, you need to bring the meatballs back to the pan and cover the dish for 10 minutes as it simmers.

- Serve onto plate and add parmesan to finish.

Keto Philadelphia Cheesesteak

Serves: 6

Ingredients:

20 ounces boneless chicken breasts

1 cup chopped onion

1 teaspoon minced garlic

1 cup diced bell pepper

4 teaspoons olive oil

4 tablespoons Worcestershire sauce

6 slices provolone cheese or queso melting cheese

1 teaspoon onion powder

Pepper to taste

1 teaspoon garlic powder

Salt to taste

Directions:

- Freeze the chicken for a while. Place chicken on your cutting board and slice into very thin slices.

- Add chicken, Worcestershire sauce, salt, pepper, onion powder, garlic powder into a bowl and mix until the chicken is well coated with the mixture.

- Place a skillet over medium heat. Add 2 teaspoons oil. When the oil is heated, add chicken and cook until underside is brown. Flip sides and cook the other side until brown.

- Remove chicken with a slotted spoon and place on a plate.

- Add 2 teaspoons oil into the same skillet. When the oil is heated, add onion, garlic and bell pepper and sauté until onion turns translucent.

- Add chicken and mix well. Remove from heat. Place cheese slices all over the chicken.

- Cover and set aside for 5 minutes.

- Serve hot.

Keto 'San Remo' Pork Chops

Serves: 2

Ingredients:

2 pork chops (loin)

1/2 teaspoon of sea-salt

1/2 teaspoon of black or white pepper

1 clove of garlic (crushed)

1 tablespoon of ground rosemary

1/4 cup of melted butter

2 tablespoons of olive oil

Directions:

- Start by preheating your oven to 350°. While it heats, season the meat with salt and pepper. Distribute evenly over both chops.

- In a bowl, combine the rosemary, garlic and

butter. Add a tablespoon of the olive oil, too.

- Using a pan or skillet which is oven-proof, heat one tablespoon of olive oil over a strong heat.

- Sear the pork chops for 3 minutes on each side. Now coat the chops with the butter/garlic sauce.

- Place the pan in the oven and let it cook for 12 minutes.

- Serve dish and use the rest of the sauce over the cooked pork chops.

Ranch Chicken with Bacon

Serves: 2

Ingredients:

2 chicken breasts, skinless, boneless

1 teaspoon ranch seasoning

2 slices thick-cut bacon

Freshly ground pepper to taste

Salt to taste

1 tablespoon chopped chives

¾ cup shredded mozzarella cheese

Directions:

- Place a skillet over medium heat. Add bacon and cook until it becomes crisp. Remove and place on a plate lined with paper towels. When cool enough to handle, crumble and set aside.

- Retain about a tablespoon of cooked fat from the skillet and discard the rest.

- Season the chicken with salt and pepper and place in the pan. Cook until golden brown and cooked through on both sides.

- Lower the heat and season with ranch seasoning. Sprinkle mozzarella on top. Cover and cook until cheese melts.

- Turn off the heat. Garnish with bacon and chives and serve.

Spicy Sausage and Cabbage Skillet

Serves: 2

Ingredients:

2 spicy Italian chicken sausages, discard casings, chopped

¾ cup shredded purple cabbage

¾ cup green cabbage, shredded

1 tablespoon coconut oil

1 tablespoon chopped fresh cilantro

¼ cup chopped onion

1 slice Colby Jack cheese

Salt to taste

Directions:

- Place a large skillet over medium–high heat. Add oil. When the oil melts, add onion and cabbage and sauté until slightly tender.

- Add sausages and cook for about 7-8 minutes.

- Place cheese slices on top and cover with a lid. Remove from heat. Let it sit for a few minutes for the cheese to melt.

- Sprinkle cilantro and serve hot.

Roasted Chicken Stacks

Serves: 4

Ingredients:

4 small chicken breasts or chicken breast cutlets

4 slices prosciutto

1 ½ teaspoons salt or to taste

1 ½ teaspoons Italian herb blend

3 tablespoons avocado oil

1 savoy cabbage, shredded

2 ½ tablespoons coconut flour

Pepper to taste

6-7 tablespoons bone broth

Directions:

- Add coconut flour, herbs and seasonings into a plastic bag and shake until well combined.

- Place chicken in it and turn the bag around a few times until chicken is well coated.

- Grease a baking sheet with oil.

- Make 4 heaps of the cabbage on the baking sheet. Season with salt. Trickle some oil on each heap.

- Top with a piece of chicken on each heap. Place a slice of prosciutto on each piece of chicken. Pour remaining oil on each heap.

- Roast in a preheated oven at 400 ° F for about 30 minutes.

- Pour broth all around the heaps in the pan. Roast for 8-10 minutes.

- Remove the stacks with a spatula. Remove one

stack at a time and place on serving plates.

- Serve hot.

Buffalo Skillet Chicken

Serves: 2

Ingredients:

½ tablespoon extra-virgin olive oil

½ teaspoon garlic powder

Freshly ground pepper to taste

1 clove garlic, peeled, minced

Cayenne pepper to taste

A handful fresh chives, chopped, to garnish

2 boneless chicken breasts

Kosher salt to taste

1 tablespoon butter

½ cup buffalo sauce

4 slices muenster cheese

Directions:

- Place a skillet over medium flame. Add oil. When the oil is heated, add garlic and sauté for a few seconds until aromatic. Add buffalo sauce and cayenne pepper and mix well.

- When it begins to simmer, add chicken and coat it well with the sauce.

- Place 2 slices Muenster cheese on each piece of chicken. Cover the skillet with a lid. Cook for a few minutes until chicken is tender.

- Sprinkle chives on top.

- Serve over greens of your choice.

Apple Pork Chops

Serves: 2

Ingredients:

1 tablespoon ghee

2 boneless pork chops

1 tablespoon monk fruit sweetener

A pinch ground nutmeg

¼ teaspoon sea salt

1 chayote, peeled, chopped into ½ inch cubes

½ teaspoon ground cinnamon

½ tablespoon apple cider vinegar

Directions:

- Place a skillet over medium heat. Add ghee. When ghee melts, add pork chops and sear for 5 minutes. Flip sides and sear for 5 minutes.

- Add chayote, cinnamon, vinegar, salt, nutmeg and monk fruit sweetener and stir. Cook until the pork chops are cooked to the desired doneness (medium-rare or medium).

- Transfer the pork chops onto a plate. Continue cooking until chayote is cooked through and resembles cooked apples.

- Divide the pork chops and mock apples into 2 plates and serve.

Cheesy Bacon Butternut Squash

Serves: 3

Ingredients:

1 pound butternut squash, peeled, cut into 1 inch cubes

1 clove garlic, peeled, minced

Salt to taste

¼ pound bacon, chopped

¼ cup freshly grated parmesan cheese

1 tablespoon olive oil

1 tablespoon chopped thyme

Freshly ground pepper to taste

¾ cup shredded mozzarella cheese

A handful of fresh parsley, to garnish

Directions:

- Place butternut squash in a baking dish. Drizzle

oil over it. Sprinkle salt, pepper, garlic and thyme and toss well.

- Top with bacon.

- Roast in a preheated oven at 425 ° F for about 30 minutes or until tender.

- Sprinkle mozzarella cheese and Parmesan cheese on top. Bake until cheese melts.

- Remove from the oven and cool for 5 minutes.

Sprinkle parsley on top and serve.

Italian Parmesan Crusted Pork Cutlets

Serves: 3

Ingredients:

3 pork cutlets

¼ cup parmesan cheese, grated

¼ cup Italian dressing

1-2 tablespoons Italian seasoning or to taste

Directions:

- Add Italian dressing into a bowl. Add Italian seasonings and stir.

- Place cheese in another bowl.

- Place a large frying pan on medium heat.

- First, dip the cutlets in the Italian dressing.

- Shake to drop off excess dressing.

- Next dredge in cheese, and place in it the pan.
Cook on both sides until brown and cooked to the
desired doneness.

- Serve hot.

Egg Roll Bowl

Serves: 3

Ingredients:

½ pound ground pork

1 small onion, thinly sliced

½ head cabbage, thinly sliced (thin and long strips)

1 clove garlic, minced

1 green onion, sliced

½ tablespoon sesame oil

1 tablespoon chicken broth or water

½ teaspoon ground ginger

2 tablespoons liquid aminos or soy sauce

Salt to taste

Pepper to taste

Directions:

- Place a pan or wok over medium flame. Add pork and cook until brown. Crumble it with a spatula as it cooks.

- Add sesame oil into the pan. Mix well with the pork. Add onions and stir. Sauté until the onions are tender.

- Add soy sauce, ginger and garlic and stir.

- Add cabbage and stir. Add broth and sauté for a couple of minutes.

- Add salt and pepper and stir. Remove from heat. Divide into 3 bowls. Garnish with green onions and stir.

Lamb Kofta Kebabs

Serves: 4

Ingredients:

1 pound ground grass-fed lamb

1 inch fresh turmeric, peeled, grated + extra to garnish

1 cup finely chopped parsley + extra to garnish

½ teaspoon salt or to taste

Directions:

- Add lamb, parsley and turmeric into the food processor and process until well combined. Make 8 equal portions.

- Take 8 wooden kebab skewers. Shape kebabs around skewers (1 portion per skewer)

- Sprinkle salt on the outside of the kebabs.

- Place a sheet of foil on a baking sheet. Place a grilling rack on the baking sheet.

- Lay the kebabs on the grill.

- Grill in a preheated oven for about 20 minutes. Turn the skewers a few times while grilling.

- Remove the kebabs from the skewers and place on a plate. Sprinkle turmeric and parsley on top and serve.

Creamy Cauliflower and Ground Beef Skillet

Serves: 2

Ingredients:

1 tablespoon ghee

1 clove garlic, chopped

½ pound lean ground beef

Freshly cracked pepper to taste

¼ cup keto-friendly mayonnaise + 2 tablespoons extra to top

2 tablespoons toasted sunflower seed butter

½ teaspoon fish sauce

2 large eggs

¼ ripe avocado, peeled, diced

½ tablespoon apple cider vinegar

2 tablespoons chopped onions

2 jalapeños peppers, sliced, divided

½ teaspoon Himalayan salt

½ pound grated cauliflower

¼ cup water

½ tablespoon coconut aminos

½ teaspoon ground cumin

A handful of fresh parsley, chopped

Directions:

- Place a cast iron skillet or a heavy-bottomed skillet over medium-high heat.

- Add ghee. When ghee melts, add onion, garlic and half the jalapeño pepper and sauté for a few minutes until slightly soft.

- Stir in beef, pepper and salt and cook until brown. Break it simultaneously as it cooks.

- Reduce heat to medium-low. Stir in the cauliflower and sauté for a couple of minutes.

- Add mayonnaise, sun butter, water, coconut aminos, and cumin, and fish sauce into a small bowl and whisk well. Pour into the skillet and mix well. Sauté until slightly dry.

- Turn off the heat. Make 2 cavities (big enough for an egg to fit in) in the mixture. Crack an egg into each of the cavities. Season with salt and pepper. Sprinkle the remaining jalapeños pepper slices over it.

- Transfer the skillet into a preheated oven. Broil for 8-10 minutes until the eggs are cooked to the desired doneness.

- Meanwhile, mix together in a bowl, 2 tablespoons mayonnaise and apple cider vinegar. Drizzle over the skillet.

- Top with avocado and parsley. Pierce the egg

yolks and serve right away.

Spinach Mozzarella Stuffed Burgers

Serves: 8

Ingredients:

3 pounds ground chuck

Pepper to taste

4 cups firmly packed fresh spinach

4 tablespoons grated parmesan cheese

1 cup shredded mozzarella cheese

2 teaspoons salt or to taste

Directions:

- Add beef, salt and pepper into a bowl and mix well. Divide the mixture into 8 equal portions and shape into patties of about ½ inch thickness. Chill for 30 minutes.

- Meanwhile, place a saucepan over medium-high

heat. Add spinach and cook until it wilts. Drain off the cooked liquid and set aside to cool.

- Squeeze the spinach of excess moisture and place on your cutting board. Chop into smaller pieces and add into a bowl.

- Add mozzarella cheese and Parmesan cheese and mix well.

- Divide the mixture into 8 equal portions and place one portion in the middle of each of the patties. Bring together the edges and press the edges together to seal. Reshape into patties.

- Place a grill pan over medium-high heat. Place the burger on the grill and cook for 5-6 minutes. Flip sides and cook the other side for 5-6 minutes. Alternately, you can grill or broil the burgers. The internal temperature of the cooked burger should be 165 ° F when checked with a meat thermometer.

- Serve as it is or with keto-friendly toppings.

Jalapeño Cheddar Stuffed Burgers

Serves: 8

Ingredients:

3 ½ pounds lean turkey or beef

Salt to taste

Pepper to taste

4 ounces cheddar cheese, shredded

2 fresh jalapeños, deseeded if desired, chopped

¼ cup finely minced onion

½ cup cream cheese

½ teaspoon garlic powder

2 tablespoons olive oil

Keto-friendly toppings of your choice

Directions:

- Add cream cheese, garlic powder, cheddar cheese and jalapeño into a bowl and stir. Divide into

8 equal portions.

- Add the meat you are using, onion, salt and pepper into a bowl and mix well.

- Divide the mixture into 8 equal portions. Shape into patties.

- Place one portion of the cream cheese mixture in the middle of each of the patties. Bring together the edges and press the edges together to seal. Re-shape into patties.

- Place a grill pan over medium-high heat. Place the burger on the grill and cook for 5-6 minutes. Flip sides and cook the other side for 5-6 minutes. Alternately you can grill or broil the burgers in an oven. The internal temperature of the cooked burgers should be 165 ° F when checked with a meat thermometer.

Taco Casserole

Serves: 3

Ingredients:

½ tablespoon extra-virgin olive oil

1 pound ground beef

Freshly ground pepper to taste

½ jalapeño, finely chopped, to garnish

1 cup shredded Mexican cheese

½ cup sour cream, to serve (optional)

1 small onion, chopped

Kosher salt to taste

1 tablespoon keto friendly taco seasoning

3 large eggs, lightly beaten

1 tablespoon chopped fresh parsley, to garnish

Directions:

- Place a skillet over medium flame. Add oil. When the oil is heated, add onion and sauté until translucent.

- Stir in beef, salt and pepper. Break it simultaneously as it cooks.

- Cook until the meat is not pink anymore.

- Add jalapeño and taco seasoning and sauté for a minute or so until aromatic.

- Turn off the heat. Discard fat in the pan. Let it cool for a while.

- Add eggs into a bowl and whisk well. Transfer the meat into the bowl of eggs and mix well.

- Transfer into a baking dish. Spread it evenly. Top with cheese.

- Bake in a preheated oven at 350 ° F for about 30 minutes or until set.

- Drizzle sour cream on top. Sprinkle parsley and jalapeño and serve.

Cheesy Kale Casserole

Serves: 8

Ingredients:

2 pounds lean ground beef

2 teaspoons kosher salt or to taste

2 teaspoons garlic powder

1 teaspoon pepper powder

2 teaspoons onion powder

20 ounces fresh kale, discard hard ribs and stems, chopped

2 teaspoons dried oregano

8 ounces mozzarella, shredded

4 tablespoons olive oil

4 cups keto-friendly marinara sauce

Directions:

- Place an ovenproof dish over medium heat.

Add oil. Once the oil is hot, add beef and cook until it is not pink anymore. Break it simultaneously as it cooks.

- Add onion powder, garlic powder, salt, pepper and oregano and stir.

- Add kale and stir. Cook until it wilts.

- Add marinara sauce and heat thoroughly. Add half the mozzarella and stir.

- Remove from heat. Sprinkle remaining mozzarella on top.

- Set the oven to broiler mode and preheat the oven.

- Transfer the dish into the oven. Broil for a couple of minutes, until cheese melts

- Remove from the oven. Cool for 5 minutes and serve.

Taco Stuffed Avocados

Serves: 2

Ingredients:

2 ripe avocados, halved, pitted

½ tablespoon extra-virgin olive oil

½ pound ground beef

Salt to taste

1/3 cup shredded Mexican cheese

¼ cup quartered grape tomatoes

Juice of ½ lime

1 small onion, chopped

½ packet taco seasoning

Freshly ground pepper to taste

¼ cup shredded lettuce

Sour cream, to drizzle

Directions:

- Scoop out some of the pulp of the avocado and place on your cutting board. You are left with avocado cases. Set them aside.

- Chop the scooped avocado and place in a bowl.

- Drizzle lime juice over the chopped avocado and set aside.

- Place a skillet over medium flame and add some oil. When the oil is hot, add onion and sauté until they get soft.

- Stir in the beef, salt, pepper and taco seasoning. Cook until the meat is not pink anymore. Break it simultaneously as it cooks.

- Turn off the heat. Discard the fat in the pan.

- Stuff this mixture in the avocado cases. Scatter the retained avocado, lettuce, tomato and cheese.

- Drizzle sour cream on top and serve.

Lemon Garlic Shrimp and Celeriac "Grits"

Serves: 4

Ingredients:

For lemon garlic shrimp:

20 large shrimp, peeled, deveined

Juice of 2 lemons

6 cloves garlic, minced

1 teaspoon + 2 tablespoons sea salt

A handful fresh parsley + extra to garnish

4 tablespoons pure avocado oil

1 teaspoon smoked paprika

½ teaspoon + ½ teaspoon pepper powder

Lemon wedges to serve

For Celeriac "Grits:

4 medium celeriac, trim the outer brown layer, cubed

2 tablespoons pure avocado oil

½ teaspoon pepper powder

4 cups chicken stock

2 medium onions, chopped

Sea salt or to taste

4 cloves garlic, peeled, minced

Directions:

- To make lemon garlic marinade: Add lemon juice, garlic, avocado oil, paprika, 1 teaspoon salt, paprika, parsley and ½ teaspoon pepper into a bowl. Mix well. Cover and set aside for a while for the flavors to set in.

- Place a large pot of water with remaining salt over medium heat. Add remaining pepper and stir.

When it begins to boil, add shrimp and cook until shrimp turns pink. Turn off the heat.

- Drain and add shrimp into the lemon garlic marinade. Cover with foil and set aside for 10 minutes.

- Serve shrimp over celeriac grits. Garnish with parsley and drizzle some lemon juice on top and serve.

- To make celeriac "grits": Add the celeriac to the food processor and pulse until you get corn grit like texture.

- Place a large nonstick skillet over medium-high heat. Add oil. When the oil is heated, add onions and sauté until translucent. Add garlic and sauté until fragrant.

- Add rest of the ingredients into the skillet and stir.

- Cover and cook for 10-12 minutes. Uncover and cook until most of the liquid is absorbed.

Salmon and Creamy Turmeric Veggies

Serves: 2

Ingredients:

2 tablespoons coconut oil or avocado oil

2 small cloves garlic, minced

½ tablespoon grated fresh turmeric

2 tablespoons water

 ½ tablespoon lime juice

1 ½ cups cauliflower florets

2 wild Alaskan salmon fillets (6 ounces each)

1 small onion, thinly sliced

1 ½ cups broccoli florets

 ½ tablespoon minced fresh ginger

¼ cup full fat coconut milk

Zest of ½ lemon, grated

Freshly ground pepper to taste

Salt to taste

½ tablespoon lemon juice

Directions:

- Place a large cast iron skillet over medium heat. Add oil. When the oil is heated, add onion, ginger, garlic and turmeric and sauté until golden brown in color.

- Add water, coconut milk, lemon juice and zest and stir.

- When it begins to boil, add vegetables, salt, and pepper, and mix well. Turn off the heat and cover with a lid.

- Meanwhile, place a grill pan over medium heat. Let the pan heat.

- Sprinkle salt and pepper over the salmon and rub it into it.

- Place on the grill and cook for 5 minutes. Flip sides and cook for 5 minutes.

- Serve salmon with the cooked vegetables.

Keto Meatloaf

Serves: 6

Ingredients:

1 onion

1 tablespoon of olive oil

2 1/2 chopped cloves of garlic

1 stalk of celery (chopped)

2 pounds of minced beef

1 teaspoon of chilli flakes/powder

1 cup of cheddar

1/2 cup of flour

1/4 cup of parmesan

2 medium eggs

1 teaspoon of salt

1 tablespoon of soy sauce

1/2 teaspoon of pepper

1 teaspoon of oregano

6 rashers of bacon

Directions:

- Preheat your oven to 380-400°.

- Grease a baking dish with olive oil.

- In a frying pan, heat 1 tablespoon of olive oil and cook the onion and celery together for 6 minutes.

- Mix the chilli, oregano and garlic in for one minute and allow the dish to cool.

- In a bowl, mix the cooked vegetables with the beef, cheddar, flour, parmesan, soy sauce, eggs, salt and pepper.

- Shape the mixture into a loaf and place in baking dish. The bacon rashers should then be placed on top.

- Cook the entire dish for 55 to 65 minutes. In the last ten minutes, place foil over dish.

Conclusion

As we come to the end of the book, I would like to thank you again for purchasing it and spending your time in reading through it. I hope you found this book a useful and informative read.

By now, you understand how ketosis works and the keto diet more than you did before you began. You can see why this has gained a cult following over the years. The keto diet will help you lose weight and also reap many other benefits that will help in improving your health and overall well being.

The diet is easy to follow and allows you to enjoy most of the food that other diets would probably ask you to give up. Now you can enjoy that dollop of butter without any guilt. And the best part is, you will know that you are losing weight even while you eat these fatty foods. Follow the list of keto-friendly foods given in the book to ensure you are following the keto diet requirements. Reducing carbs from your diet will play a big role in this.

Use the recipes given here to help you whip up some delicious keto-friendly meals, to begin with. Once you see the keto diet work for you, you may even recommend this keto guide to other friends or family who could use it for themselves.